My Note for You:

TO BETHANY - MOTHER OF 4 DRAGONS.
THANK YOU FOR BEING SUCH A WONDERFUL INSPIRATION TO SO
MANY MOMS AND MOMS-TO-BE!

PRECIOUS
Published by LHC Publishing 2021

Text Copyright © 2021 Y. Eevi Jones
Illustrations Copyright © 2021 Y. Eevi Jones
Cover Design by Y. Eevi Jones
Cover Art by Anna Ismagilova

Printed in the USA.

All inquiries should be directed to
www.LHCpublishing.com

ISBN-13: 978-1-952517-13-6 Paperback
ISBN-13: 978-1-952517-12-9 Hardcover

Life's Biggest Moments

PRECIOUS

For New Moms and Moms-to-Be

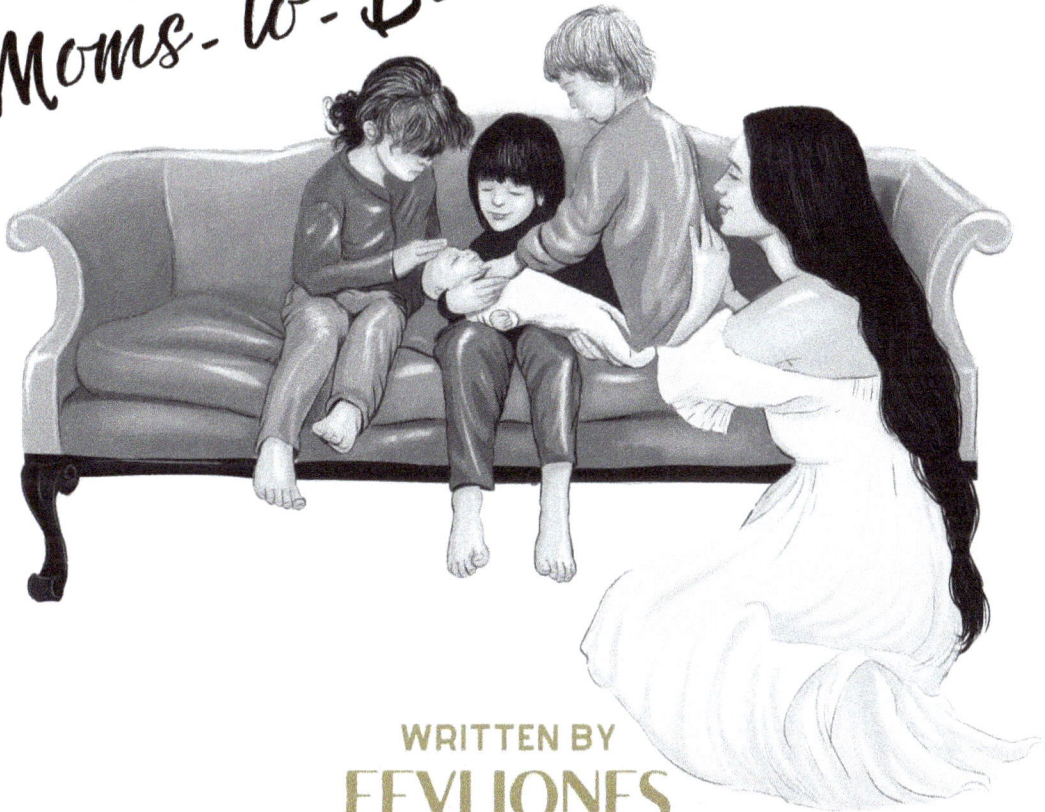

WRITTEN BY
EEVI JONES

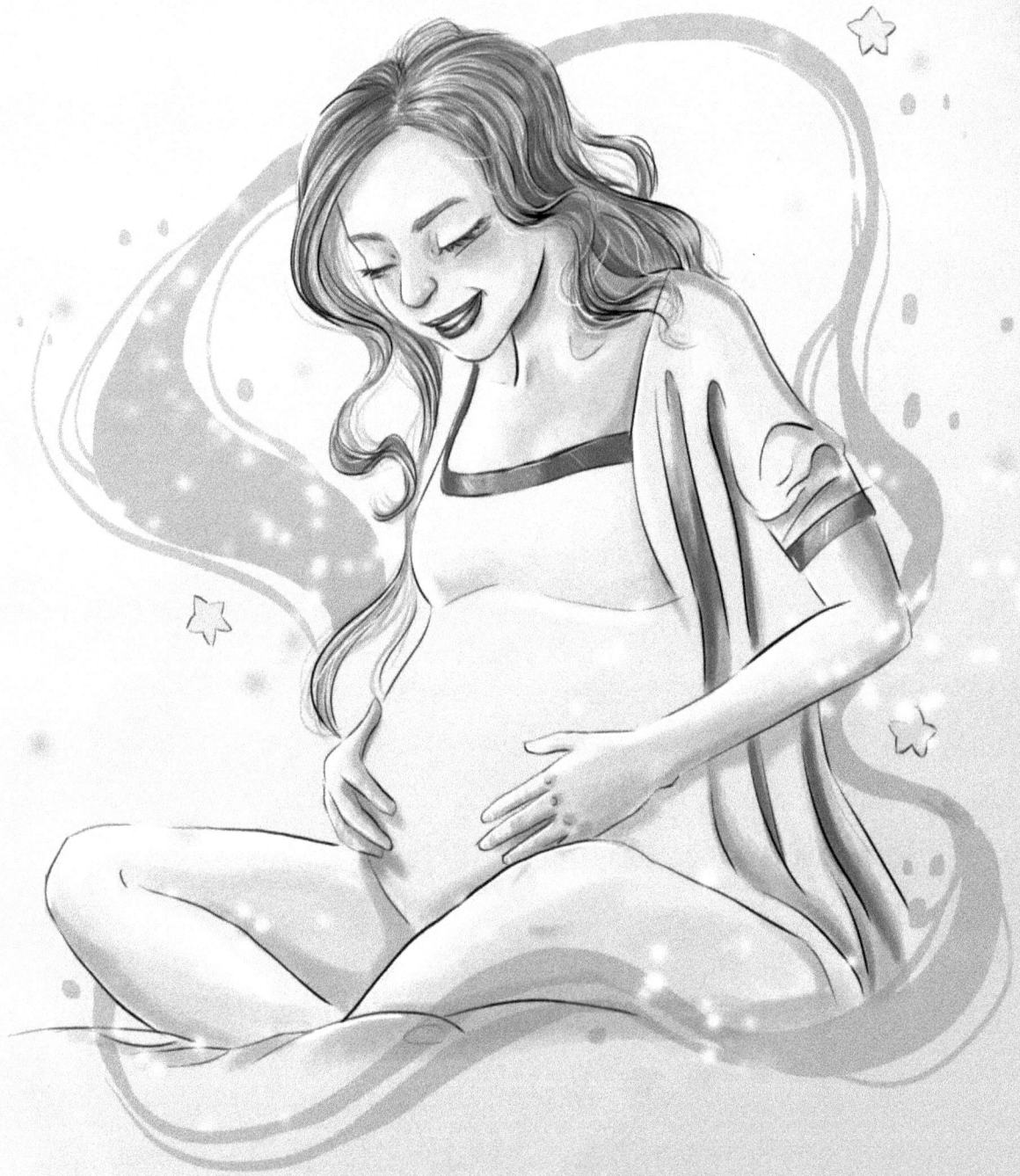

My Sweet Friend:

From the moment you hear the heart beating
to the moment you feel that first kick,
an indescribable bond - it is formed;
unbreakable and inconceivably big.

So big, it allows to endure,
providing all the strength you will need
for the months that now lie ahead,
until you both finally meet.

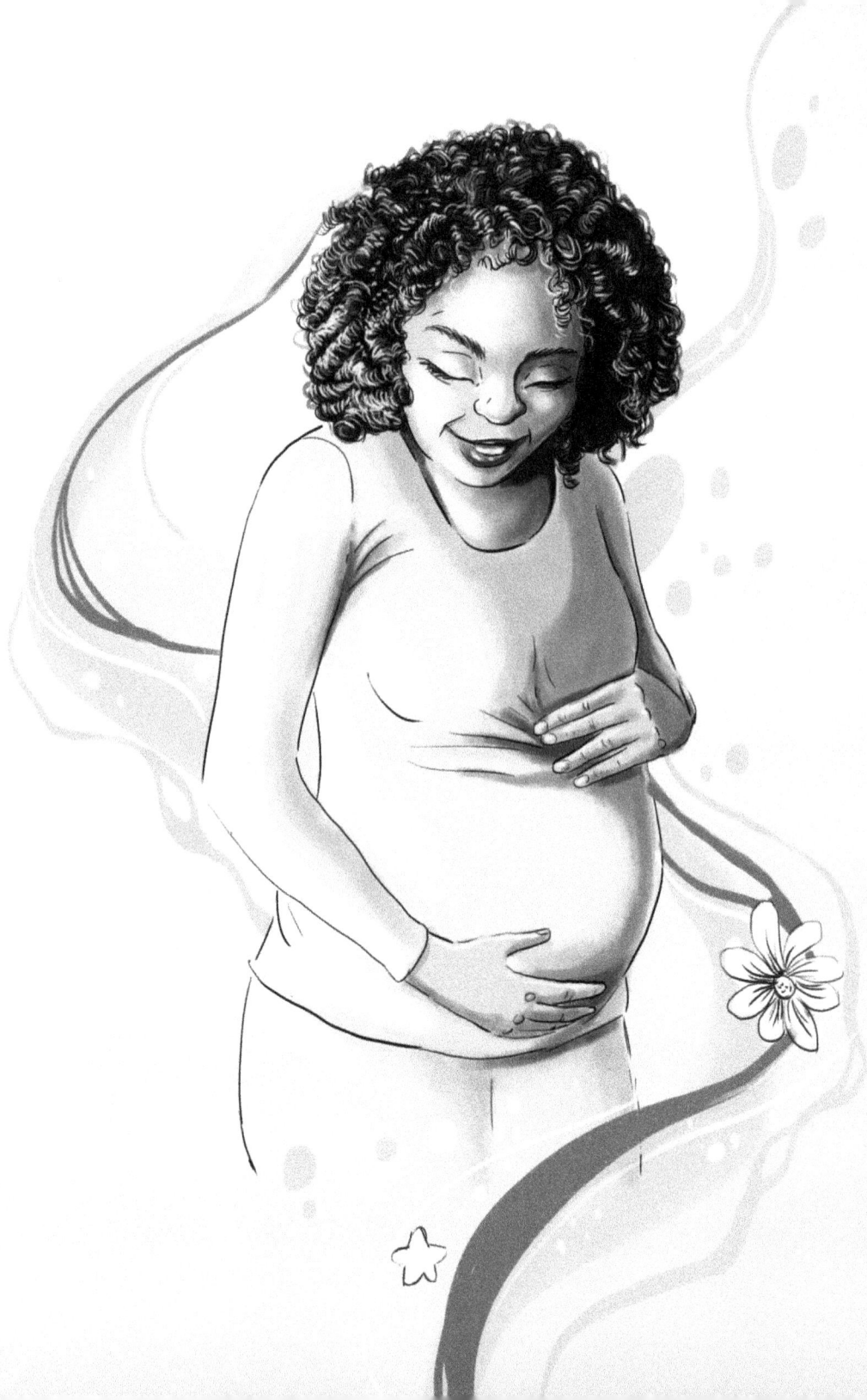

Oh what magic you've willed into being.
What marvel you've brought to this earth.
What miracle you have created,
be it through adoption, surrogacy, or birth.

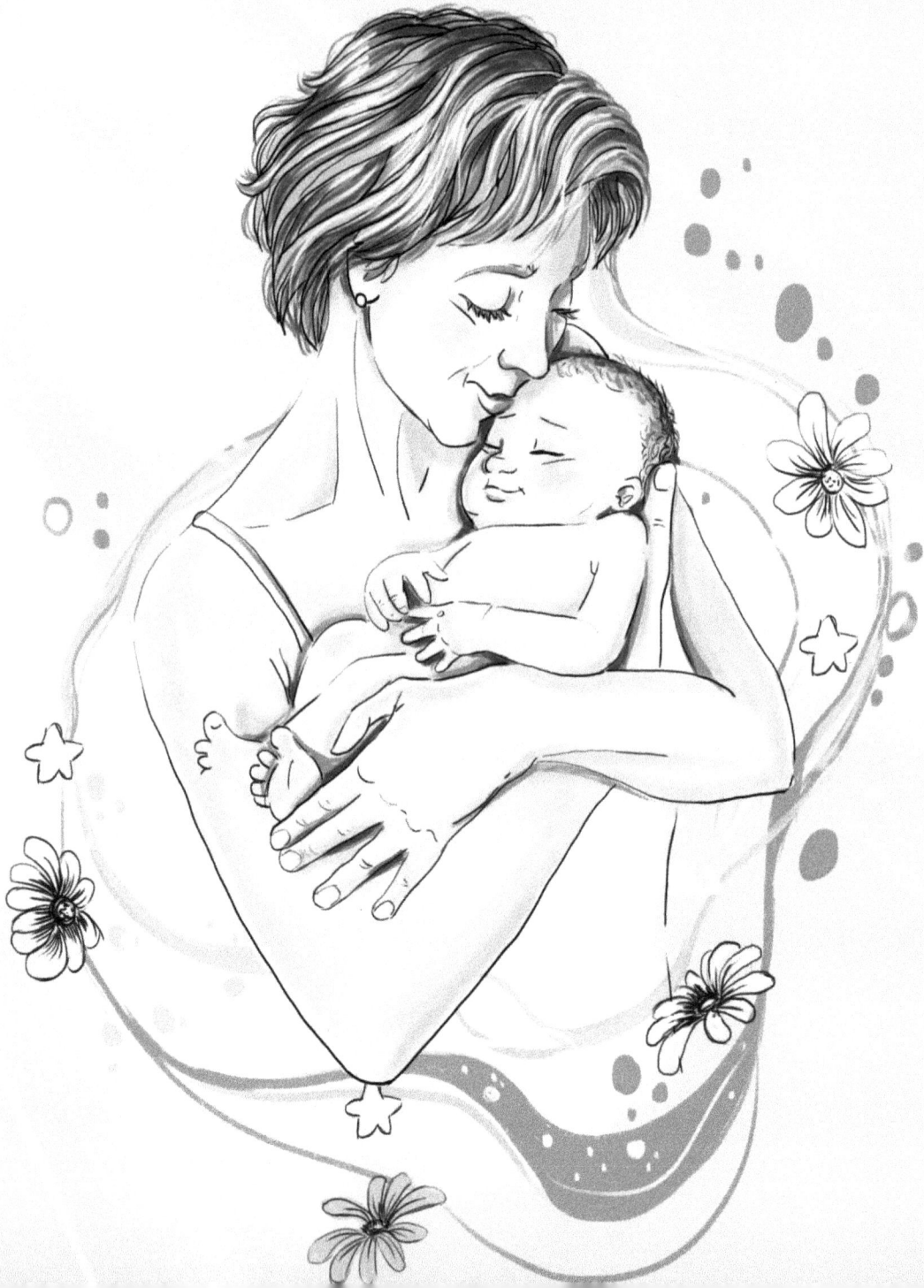

Motherhood is such a wonderful gift,
so take the new and unknown day by day;
where choices are based on what's best for you both,
no matter what others may say.

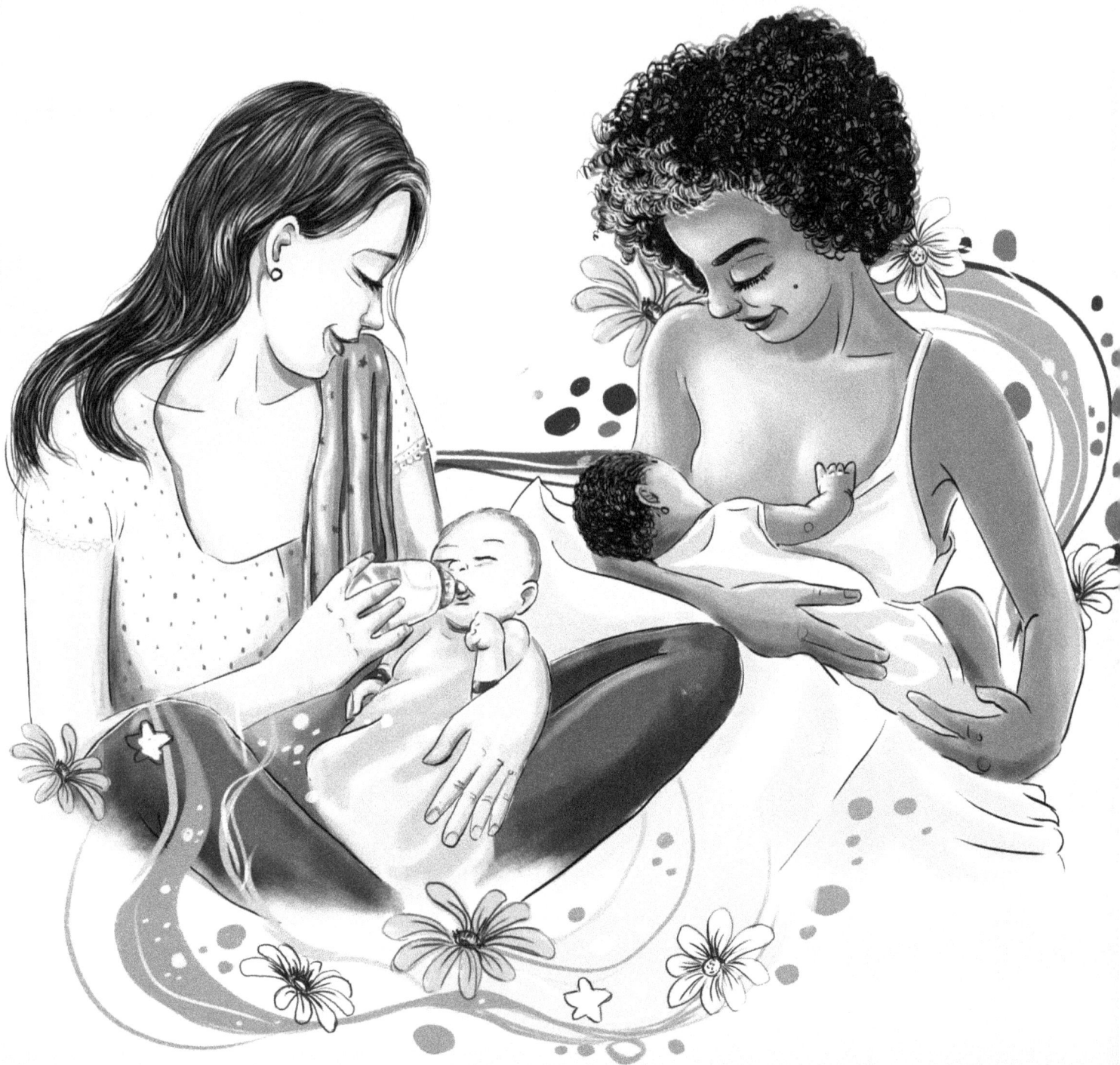

Whether bottle, breast, or a mix in between,
there is no right or wrong!
For no matter how well meaning others' advice,
in the end, the decision is yours alone.

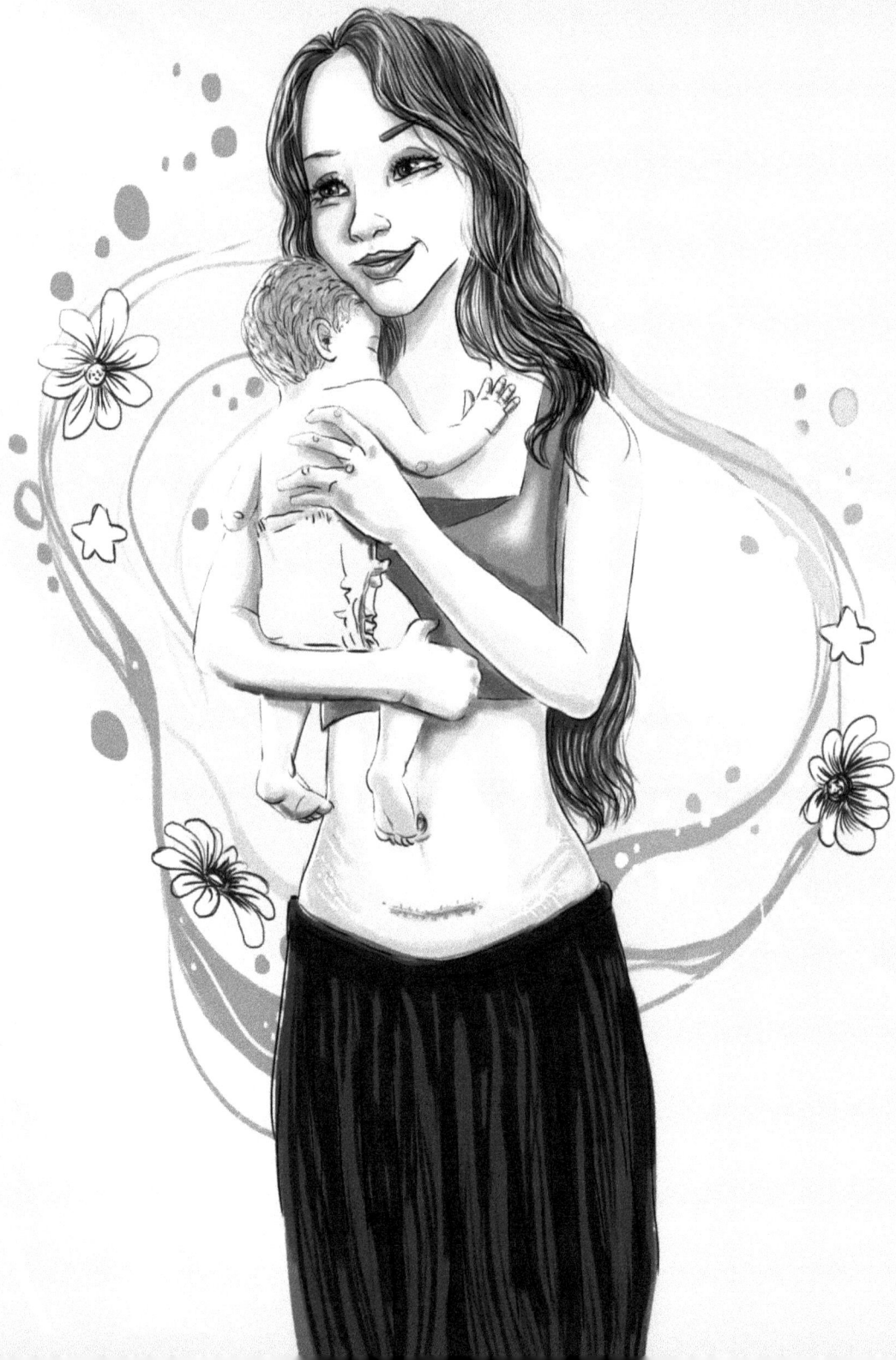

May you see your body with wonder;
filled with awe and love, never fault.
For thanks to all that it is, has become, and can do,
it nourished and grew the life you now hold.

So be gentle with yourself -
what you think, expect, deem right.
For every scar, and ounce, and mark
shows your body's strength and might.

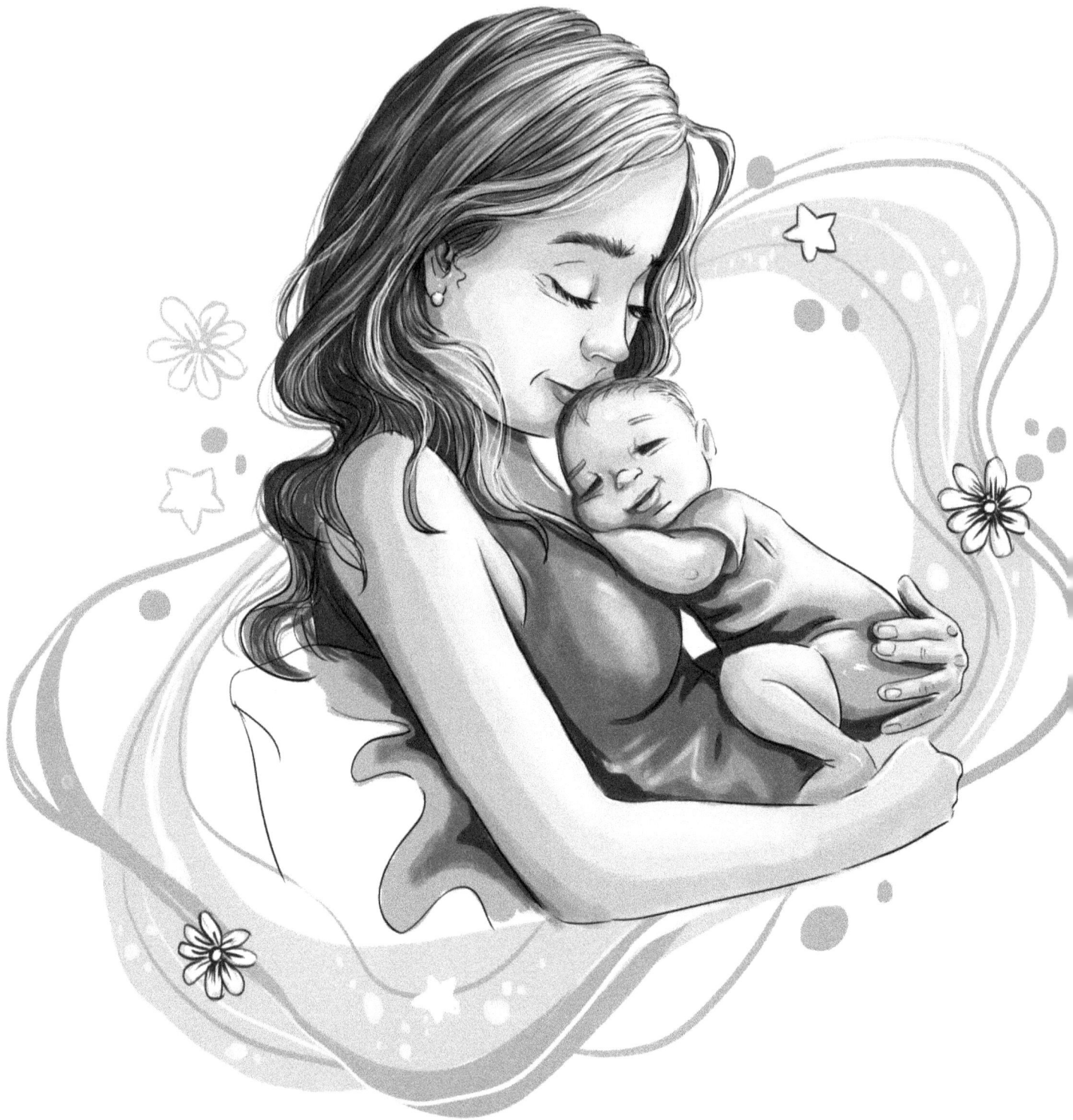

Your emotions keep you guessing,
feelings wrapped in haze and blur.
You're happy, excited, and over the moon;
yet feel scared and so insecure.

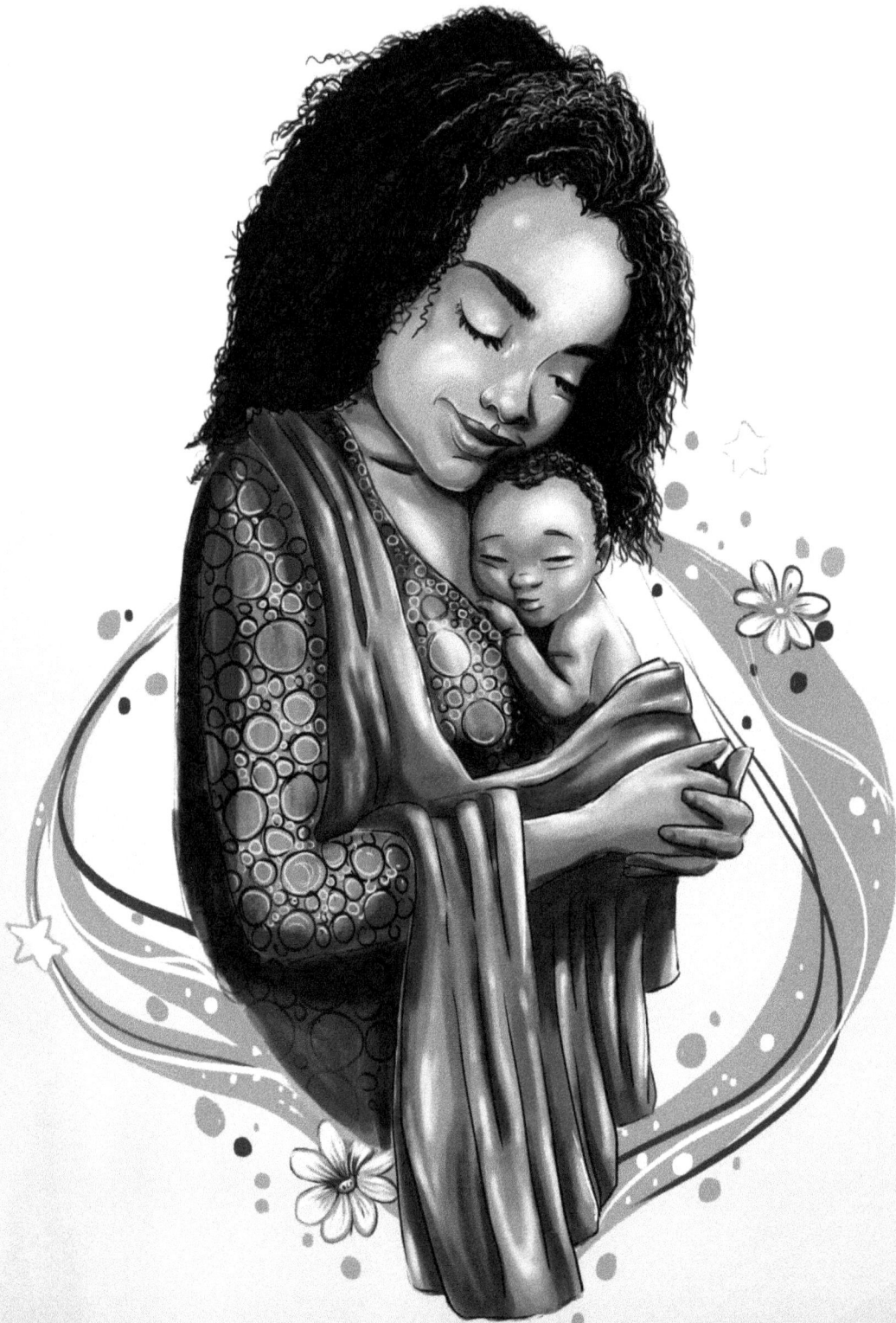

Insecure about the future;
'bout the things you yet don't know;
all the answers you don't have;
the unknown paths you now must go.

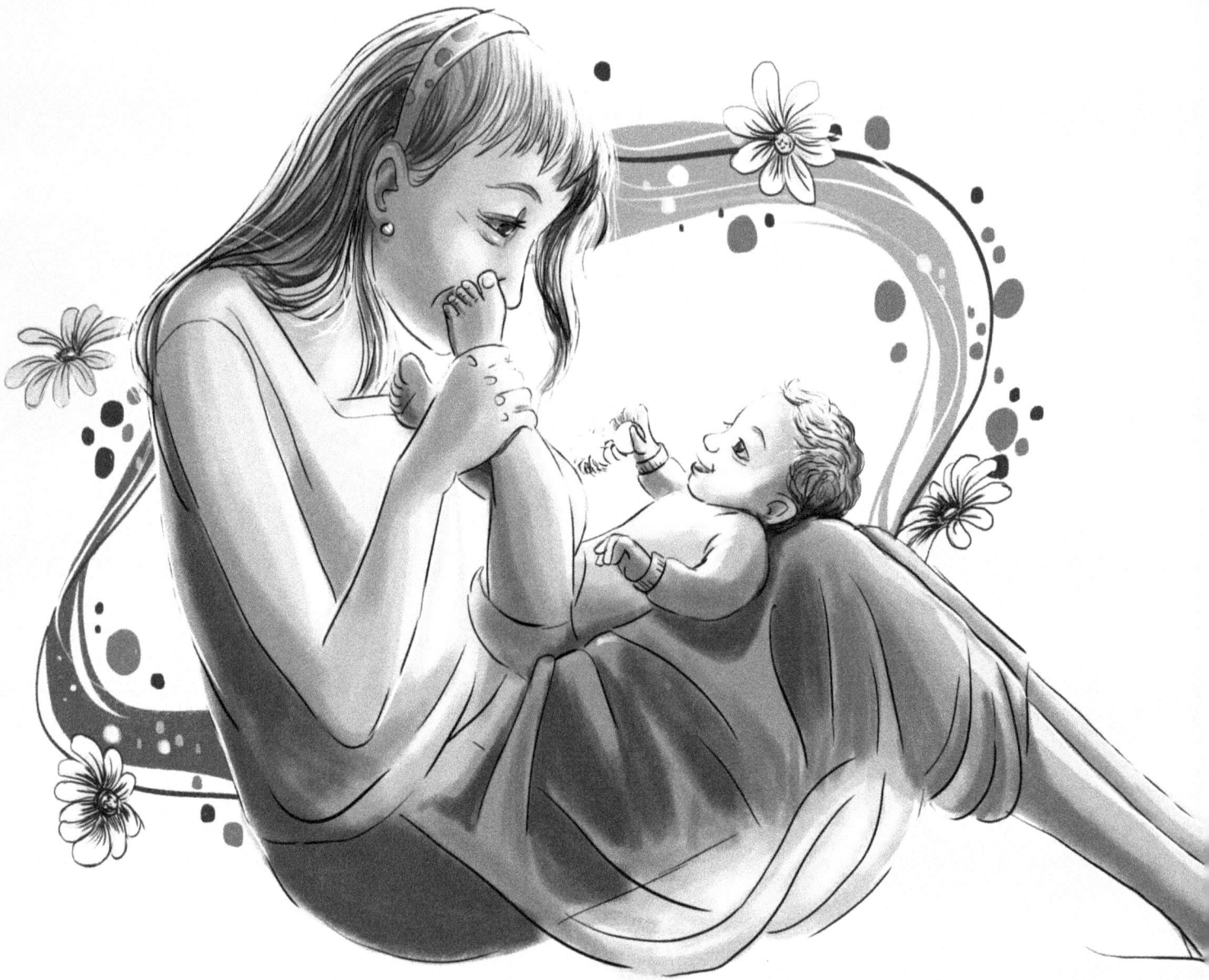

Yet no one knows what they are doing,
for there's no playbook, key, or guide.
Through trial and error we live and we learn,
and adopt what works and feels right.

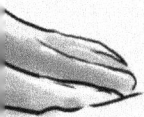

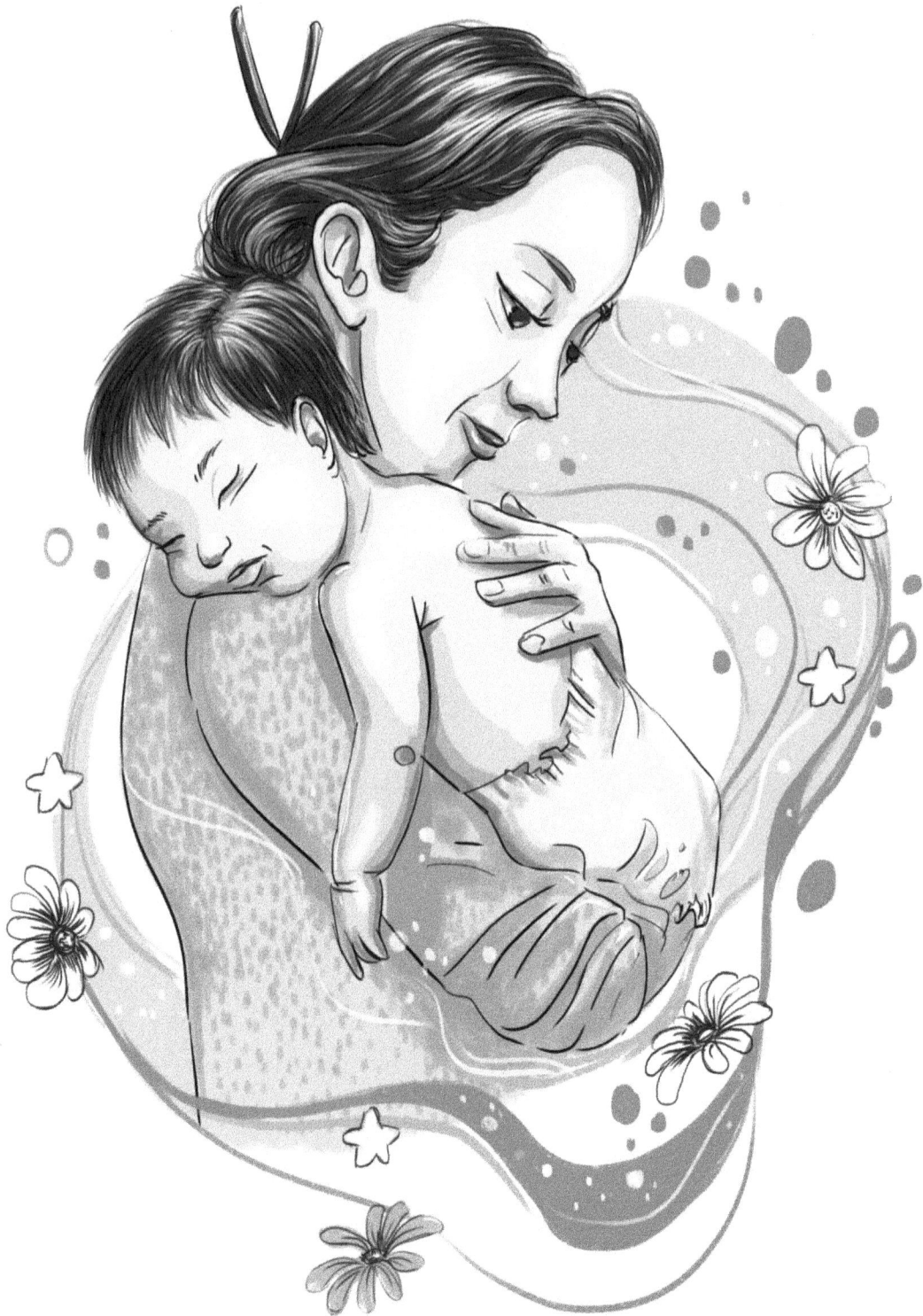

Your parenting journey will be filled with mistakes;
yet, give yourself some grace.
Both you and your baby learn new things every day.
You adjust. You grow. You embrace.

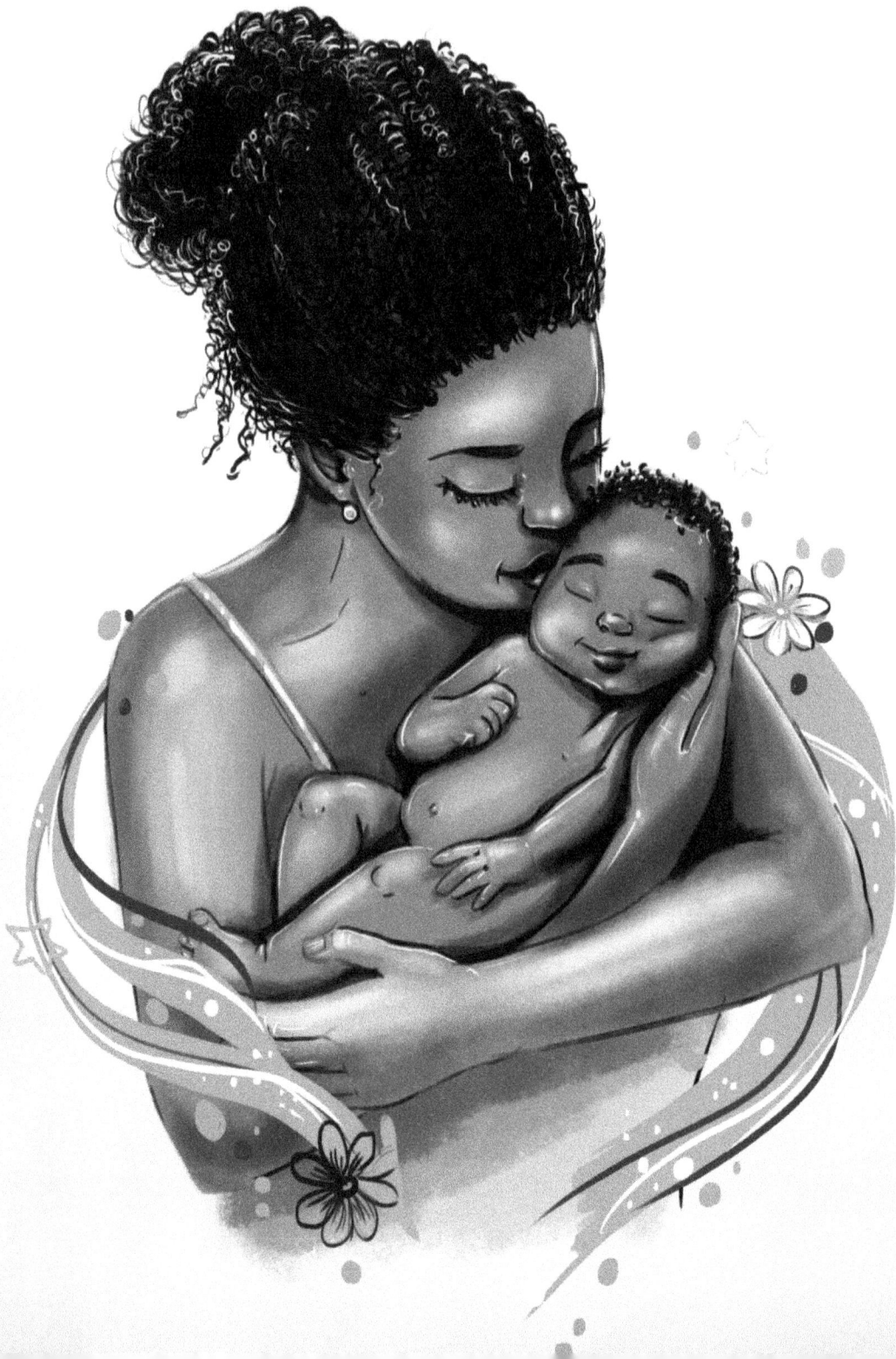

You adjust to all the changes.
You grow through all the new.
You embrace what can't be changed.
Outlast moments you feel blue.

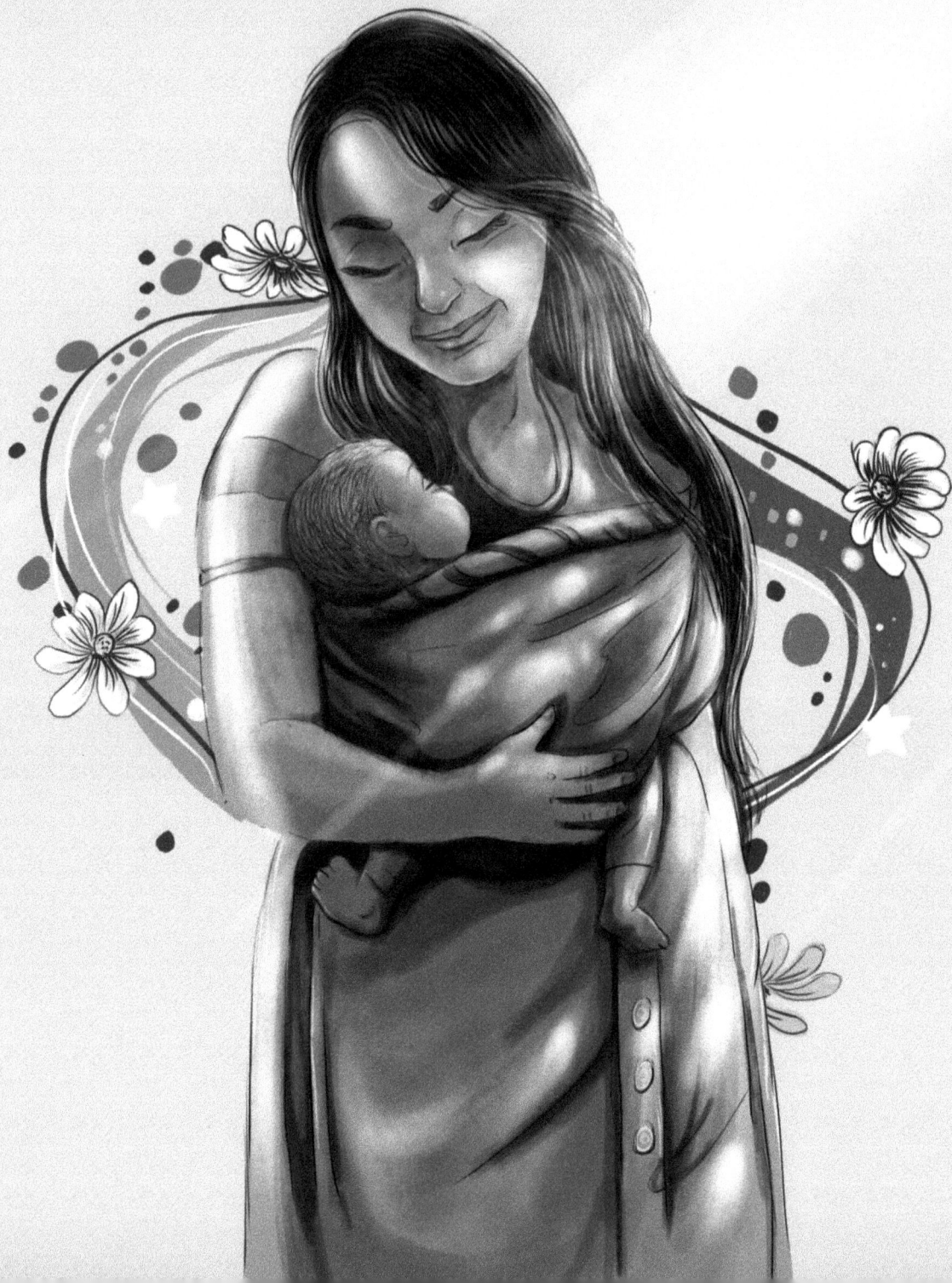

For these moments too shall pass.
Every wakeful, sleepless night
is nothing but a phase,
all with an end in sight.

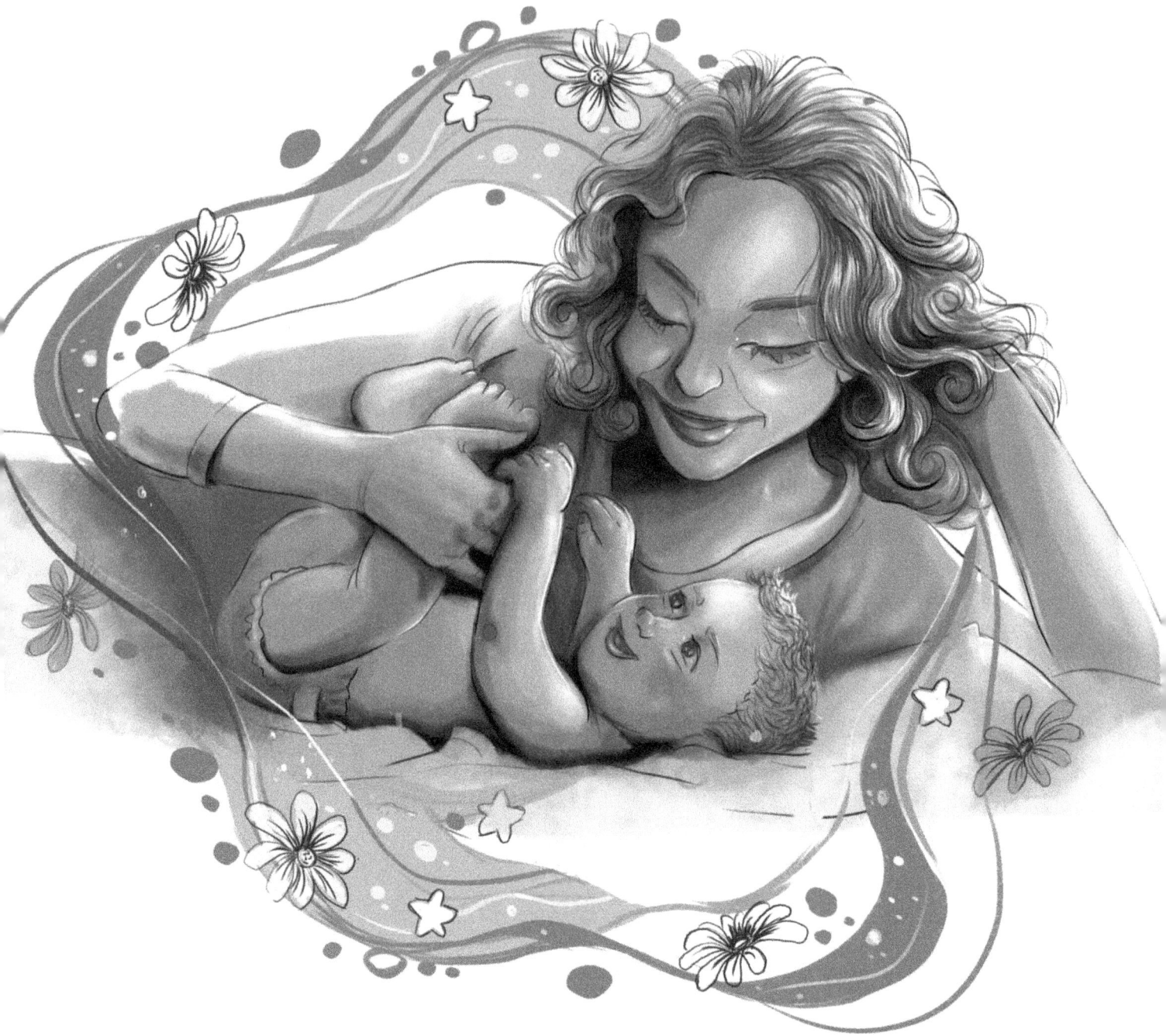

It's not the messes that will be remembered,
but the love and the bond you create.
What remains in your hearts and your minds
are the laughs and the memories made.

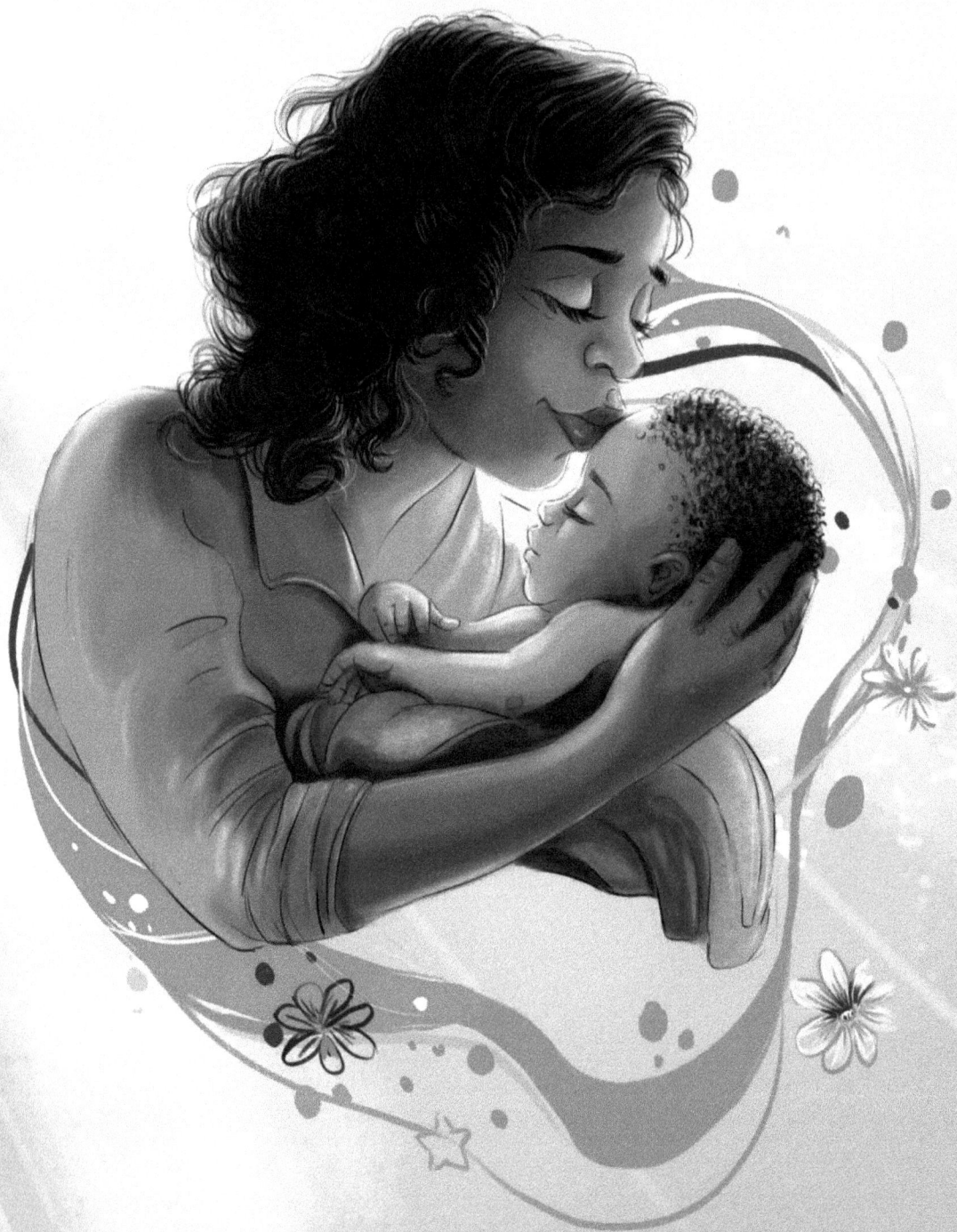

So whenever you feel like you're failing,
know that you will be okay.
For all good parents, they fear and they doubt
themselves in every which way.

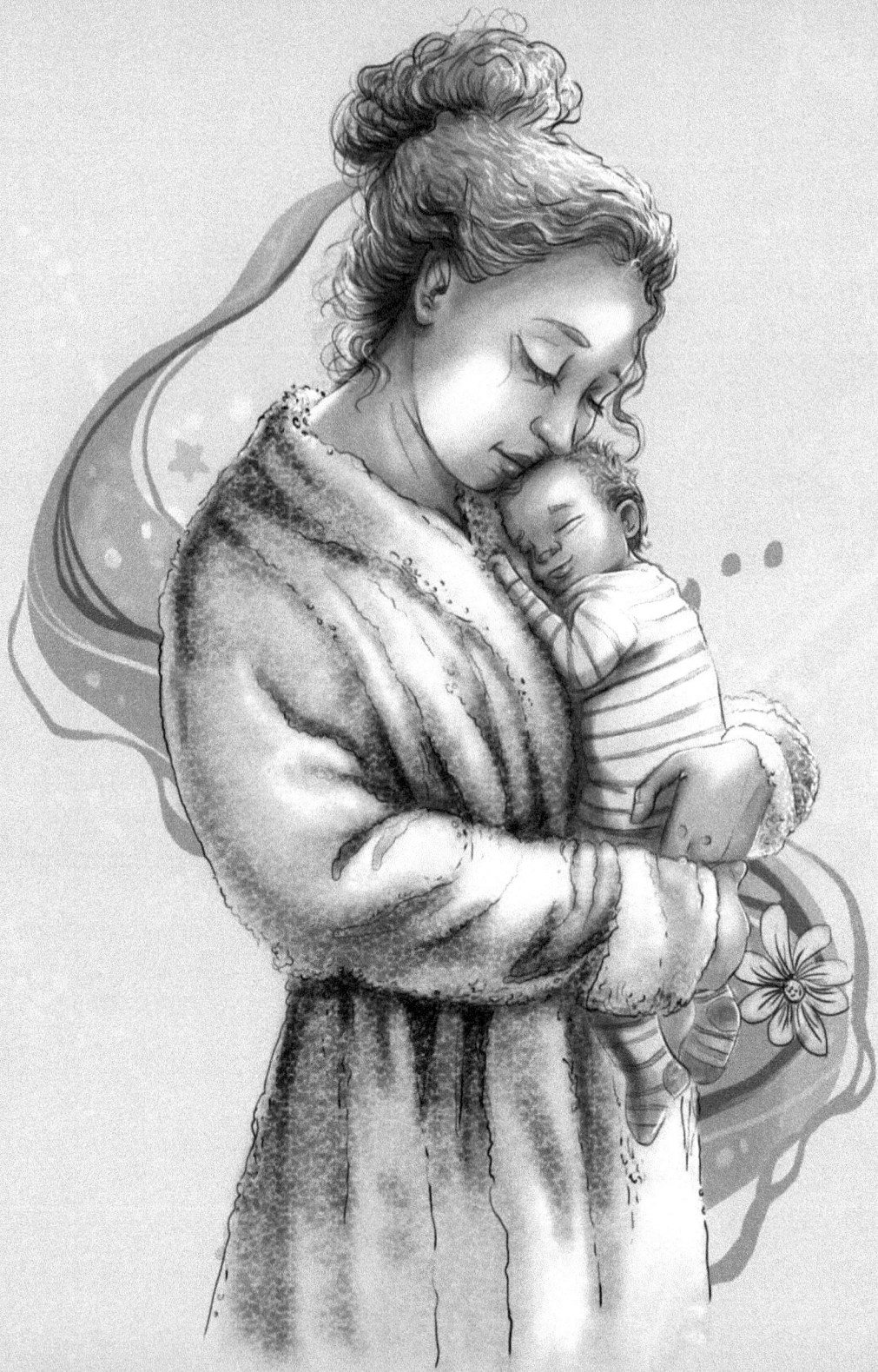

It truly takes a village,
sometimes big and sometimes small.
This is a journey not meant to be walked
on your own, with no help at all.

So be brave, ask for support.
Share your wants and what you need,
giving you the time and rest
you might lack but seek.

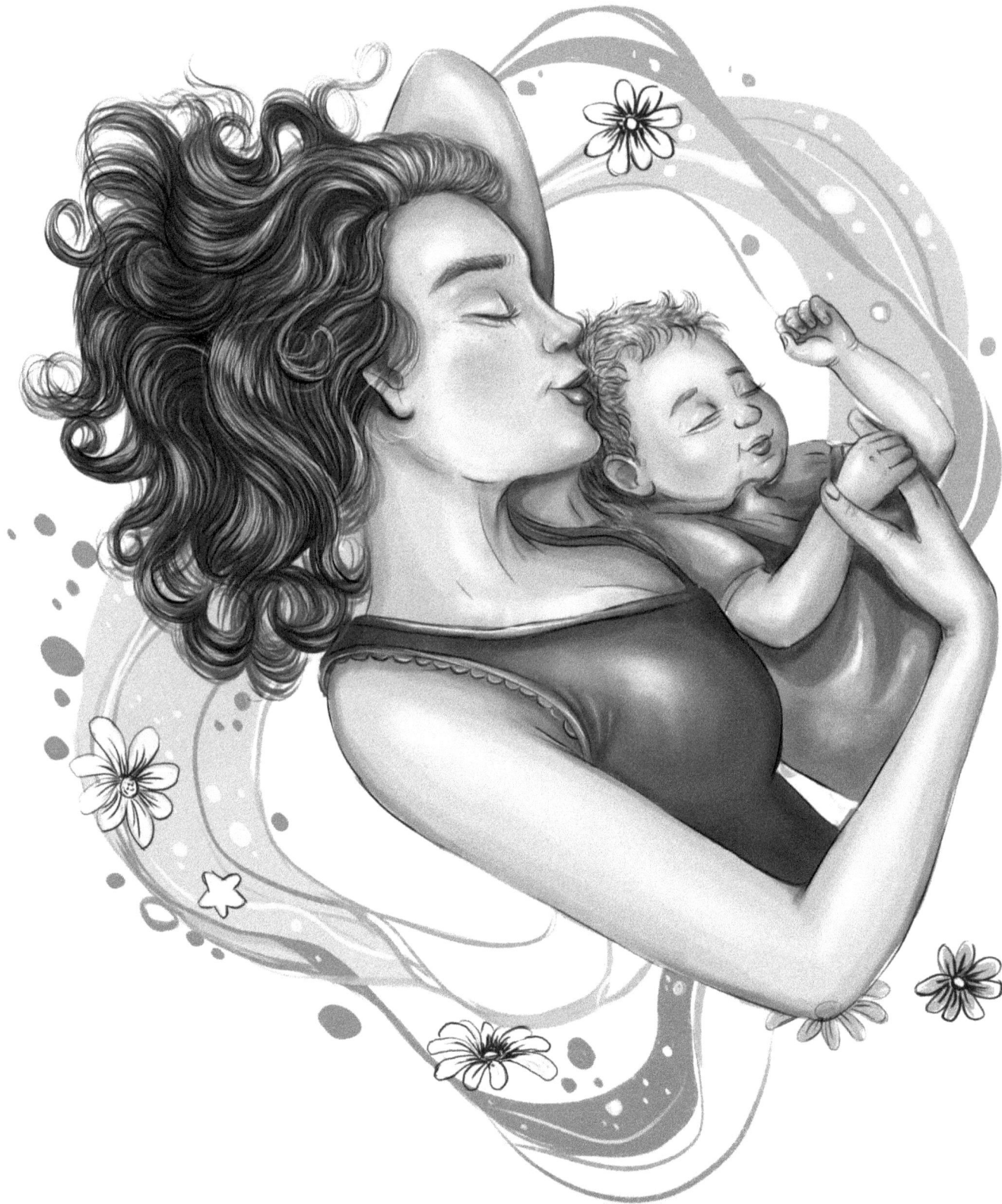

No bond is stronger in this world.
No love so true and pure.
Your heart will grow beyond a size
you've ever known before.

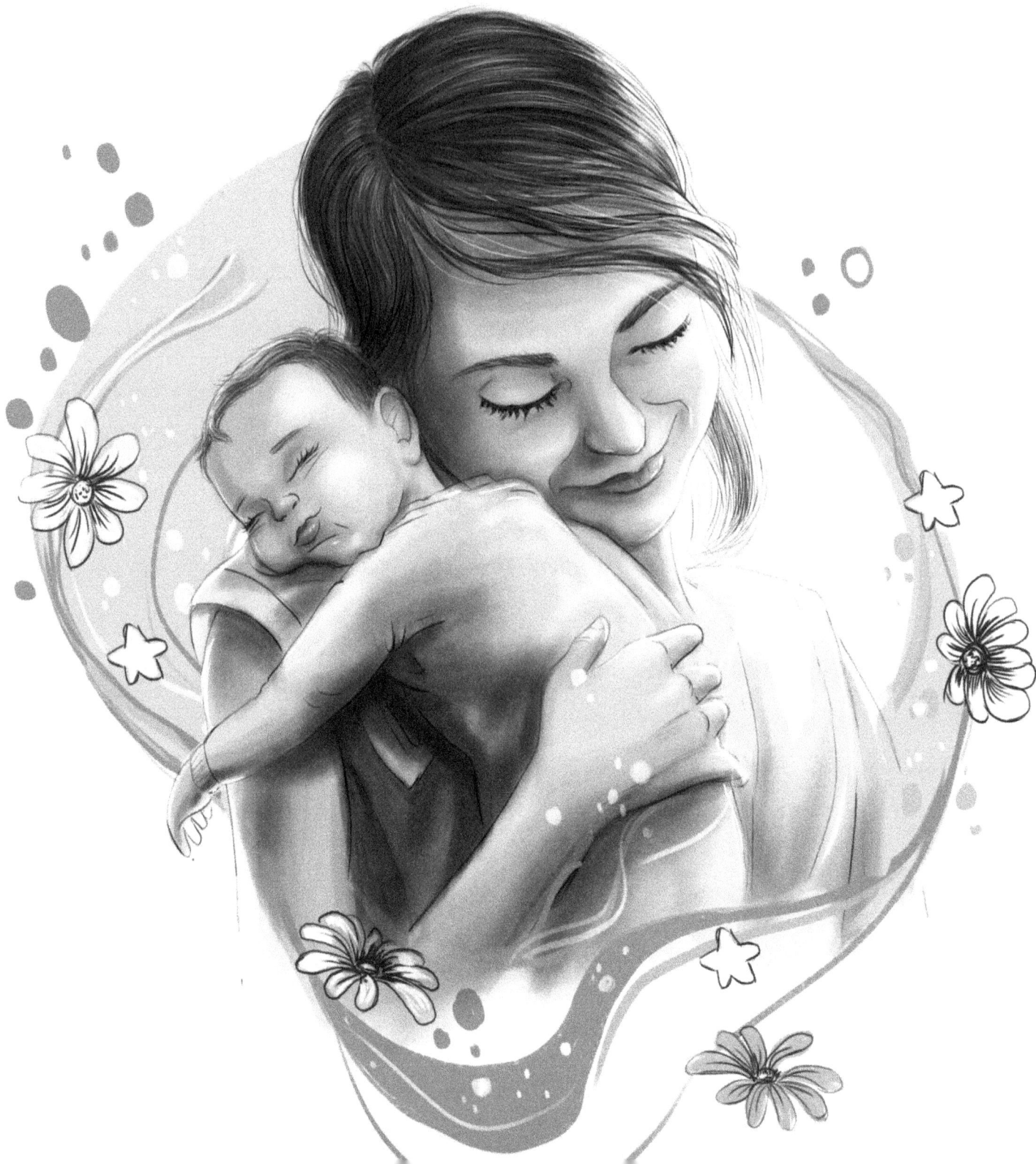

216 months –
that's all the time you get
until your baby turns 18.
So make it count, with NO regret.

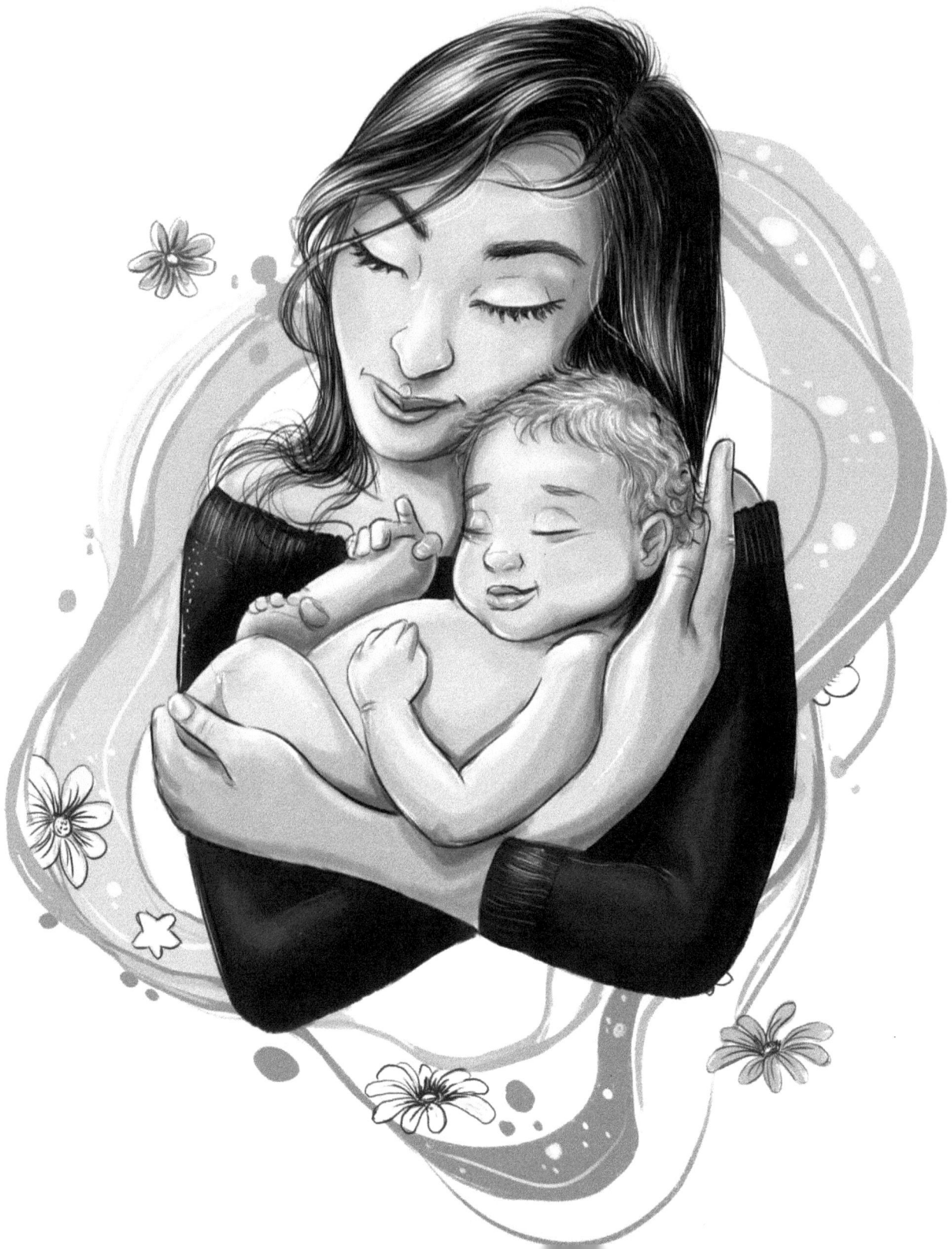

Take in every single moment;
whether messy, hard, or sweet.
For your most fulfilling life begins
the moment you both first meet.

ABOUT THE AUTHOR

Writing under a number of pen names, Eevi Jones is a USA Today & WSJ bestselling and award-winning author and ghostwriter of children's books.

Born in former East Germany to a German mother and a Vietnamese father, Eevi loves to infuse her children's books with racial diversity. She is the founder of Children's Book University where dreams really do come true. "Life's Biggest Moments" is Eevi's first series for adults.

Eevi has been featured in media outlets such as Forbes, Scary Mommy, Business Insider, Huffington Post, and Exceptional Parent Magazine, and lives near D.C. with her husband and two boys.

She can be found online at www.BravingTheWorldBooks.com.

A WORD BY THE AUTHOR

Becoming a new parent often comes with great excitement and anticipation, but also doubt and uncertainty. I hope that with this book you come to see that there are no set rules, only those you create yourself. Let this new season in your life be filled with awe and wonder, overflowing with nothing but acceptance, appreciation, and self-love.

If this book touched you in any way, it would mean the world to me if you would take a short minute to leave a heartfelt review. Thank you.

OTHER WORKS BY THIS AUTHOR

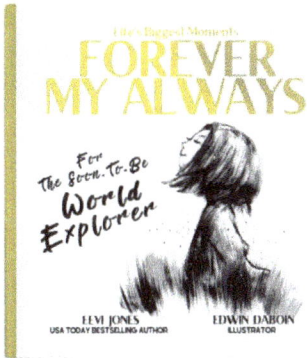

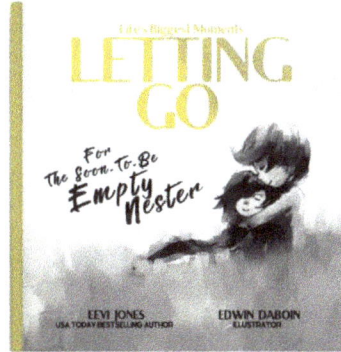

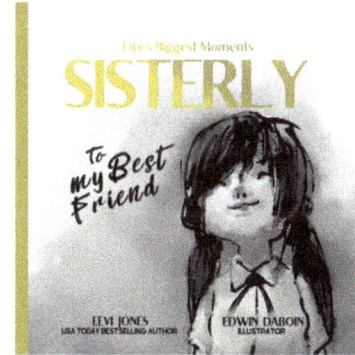

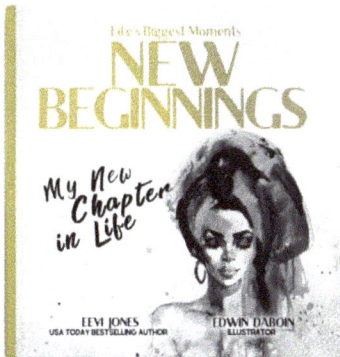

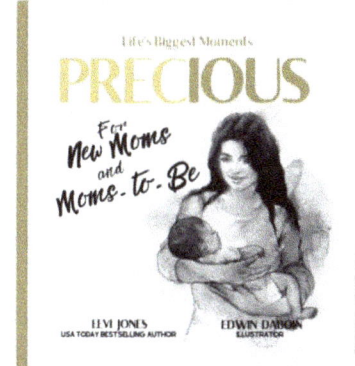

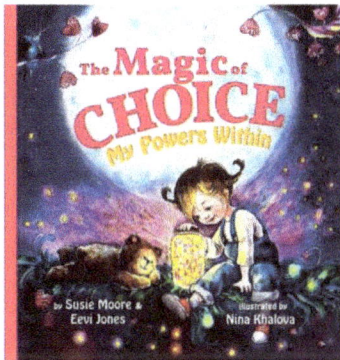

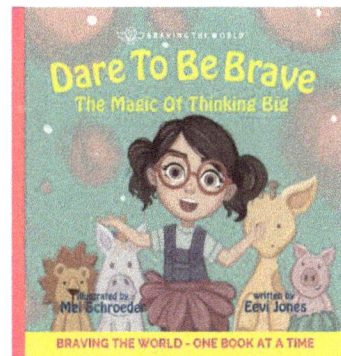

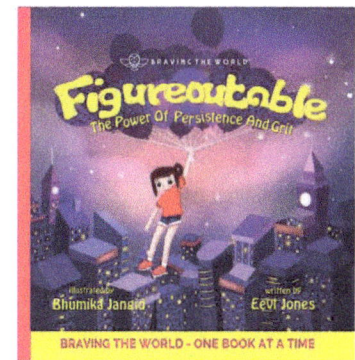

Life's Biggest Moments
FOREVER MY ALWAYS
For The Soon-To-Be World Explorer
EEVI JONES
USA TODAY BESTSELLING AUTHOR
EDWIN DABOIN
ILLUSTRATOR

Life's Biggest Moments
LETTING GO
For The Soon-To-Be Empty Nester
EEVI JONES
USA TODAY BESTSELLING AUTHOR
EDWIN DABOIN
ILLUSTRATOR

Life's Biggest Moments
SISTERLY
To my Best Friend
EEVI JONES
USA TODAY BESTSELLING AUTHOR
EDWIN DABOIN
ILLUSTRATOR

Life's Biggest Moments
NEW BEGINNINGS
My New Chapter in Life
EEVI JONES
USA TODAY BESTSELLING AUTHOR
EDWIN DABOIN
ILLUSTRATOR

BRAVING THE WORLD

Life's Biggest Moments
PRECIOUS
For New Moms and Moms-to-Be
EEVI JONES
USA TODAY BESTSELLING AUTHOR
EDWIN DABOIN
ILLUSTRATOR

The Magic of CHOICE
My Powers Within
by Susie Moore & Eevi Jones
Illustrated by Nina Khalova

BRAVING THE WORLD
Dare To Be Brave
The Magic Of Thinking Big
Illustrated by Mel Schroeder
written by Eevi Jones
BRAVING THE WORLD - ONE BOOK AT A TIME

BRAVING THE WORLD
Figureoutable
The Power Of Persistence And Grit
Illustrated by Bhumika Janaid
written by Eevi Jones
BRAVING THE WORLD - ONE BOOK AT A TIME

... AND MANY MORE

www.ingramcontent.com/pod-product-compliance
Lightning Source LLC
Chambersburg PA
CBHW041601260326

41914CB00011B/1341